Heart of a Father Love of an Husband

Secret Of A Loving Father, And A Prominent Husband

By

Tim Annex

Table of Contents

Introduction

Conclusion

Introduction

Getting Started: A Handbook for New Fathers

This guide's main goal is to assist you in understanding what it can be like to be a father, taking care of yourself and those around you, and doing your best to develop into a self-assured parent.

This book is an attempt to address the queries and worries that you will probably have when you embark on your parenthood journey. We've also included resources to help you with one of the most significant and rewarding jobs in the world: being a father! We hope this information will point you in the direction of any support and guidance you may require along the journey.

This manual draws from the experiences of thousands of fathers who have gone through this journey before you and is based on the greatest, most recent research available.

The "becoming Dad" science Your experiences as a new or soon-to-be father are the result of many centuries of evolution. What does science have to say about the needs of children and the ways in which becoming a father alters men?

Taking care of yourself: It may sound cliche, but if you don't know how to take care of yourself, how can you possibly take care of others? This chapter is all about being vulnerable with yourself, being open about how you feel about becoming a father, and figuring out how to keep your cool and concentrate on what really matters during what may be an exciting but demanding time.

assisting the biological mother of your child Regardless of your love or platonic relationship, this individual will play a significant role in your child's development and experience some very difficult times. Here, we'll concentrate on the physical journey of biological mothers and your potential support.

Taking care of your partnership with your partner: For a couple, the prenatal stage can be a minefield that either makes or breaks the relationship. This chapter covers the main issues and provides helpful advice for preserving or enhancing your relationship. We also examine your options in case something goes wrong.

Getting to know your child – Men may have trouble initiating a conversation or "engaging" with their unborn child. Here, we'll look at easy strategies to establish a solid link with your child and begin figuring out how to make everyone work in your new family.

Balancing work and home life: Dads often face pressure from family, friends, the larger community, and ourselves to be "the provider." Here, we'll examine how to manage this facet of your paternal identity and provide helpful advice on how to maximize the time you spend with your child and strike a work/life balance that will enable you to be a fully engaged father.

There are a lot of questions while getting ready to become a mom. And maybe some unsolicited counsel. and counsel that contradicts itself. And, with any luck, some really helpful guidance.

Being a parent may be a thrilling experience. It may also be mentally and physically exhausting. Your relationships are altered by it. It alters your perspective on who you are and what matters most. Raising a child alters your approach to self-care.

We had a conversation with a parenting educator on the things that new fathers should know and how to get ready for the opportunities and adjustments that come with becoming a father.

You've come to the right place if you're seeking help as a new parent or soon-to-be parent. A lot of the guidance we discussed with a writer is applicable to all parents. That encompasses all of the individuals on your parenting team, including birth parents and those who firmly identify as "dads."

Parents of all gender identities are welcome here. You're in the proper place if you're looking for help on being a new parent, rather than specific information on getting pregnant, giving birth, breastfeeding, or anything else related to your assigned sex at birth.

Greetings from the new dad club! Now let's get started!

First-time fathers: what should they know and do?
To begin with, it's admirable that you are researching fatherhood and seeking guidance. We all prefer to act as though we know more than we actually do far too often in life. And one of those things you really never know what to anticipate until you're in the midst of things, trying to figure it out, is being a parent for the first time.

However, you can become more prepared the more you read, the more you inquire, and the more you express your ideas. As someone once said:

He observes, "A lot of us weren't raised to ask these kinds of questions." "It is incredibly powerful and vital to take the time to ask questions and look for solutions. You'll be able to influence your child's life to an even larger extent the more you communicate and ask questions.

Chapter 1

<u>What Does Being A Father Entail?</u>

The traditional family and society are changing, and so is the art of parenthood. By using these constructive parenting techniques, fathers may assist their children in developing self-worth and confidence, which will help them become more involved, loving, and supportive fathers.

The types of families that exist today are becoming more and more varied. These include same-gender, blended, single-parent, single-parent, and multigenerational families. Maternal and paternal responsibilities have changed over the last thirty years due to societal transformations brought about by the increase in women working outside the house, rising divorce rates, remarriages, and mixed families.

If you ask any father today, he will most likely tell you that the interactions he has with his sons or daughters are very different from the ones he had with his own father. Men now have more alternatives for how to fulfill their responsibilities as husbands, fathers, and partners because to changes in parenting practices. Dads of today are less inclined to naturally draw instruction on his own fatherhood from his own childhood experiences. What worked effectively for his father thirty years ago would not function at all with the complex and varied issues that current fathers face, given the way that fathers' roles are continually evolving.

According to recent studies, children of warm, accepting fathers typically have higher self-esteem. A loving and supportive father-child bond promotes children's growth in terms of accomplishments, social acceptance, and personal growth. Competency is fostered in children by loving fathers who provide sensible, solid leadership without arbitrarily imposing their will.

Becoming an Involved, Caring, and Supportive Father: Parenting Advice for Dads

- **Take Time To Interact With Your Youngster.** A father's priorities are shown to his child by the way he spends his time. The moment to strengthen your bonds with your children is now, as they grow up swiftly. There are lots of enjoyable activities you can do as a family with your kids.

- **Positive Parenting And Loving Discipline.** To set reasonable boundaries rather than as a form of punishment, all children require good direction and discipline. Fathers ought to encourage positive behavior in their kids and remind them of the repercussions of their actions. Dads who punish their kids fairly and with calmness demonstrate their love for them.

- **Set An Example For Your Children.** Fathers serve as role models for their children, whether they are aware of it or not. A girl who grows up with a loving father understands what to seek for in a mate and grows up believing that boys should treat her with respect. Fathers set an example of integrity, modesty, and responsibility for their children, teaching them valuable lessons about life.

- **Get The Opportunity To Be Heard.** In order to make challenging subjects simpler for their children to grasp when they get older, fathers should start having essential conversations with their young children. Allocate time to hear your child's thoughts and concerns.

- **Act As A Teacher For Your Kids.** Teaching your kids about right and wrong and motivating them to achieve their best is part of being a good parent. Make sure your kids make wise decisions. Engaged fathers teach their kids life lessons through real-world examples.

- **Share A Meal As A Family.** Family meals are a great way to strengthen bonds within the family. It provides an opportunity for children to discuss what they are doing and would like to do. Fathers should take advantage of this opportunity to participate and listen. It gives families a routine for spending time together every day.

- **Give Your Child A Book To Read..** Fathers should make the effort to read to their children in order to develop lifelong readers in a society when television and the internet rule. When kids grow older, encourage them to read independently by starting to read to them at an early age. One of the best methods to guarantee children's lifetime literacy and opportunities for personal and professional development is to instill a love of reading in them.

- **Show Respect To Your Child's Other Parents.** Children live in a safe atmosphere when their parents treat each other with respect and show that regard to their children as well. Children are more likely to feel welcomed and valued in the father-child relationship when they witness their parents treating each other with respect.

- **Encourage Participation As Soon As Possible.** Demonstrate interest at a young age by learning about a father's responsibilities during pregnancy, adoption, and surrogacy, and by playing, holding, and gently touching your infant. Fathers who are involved provide a strong and unambiguous message: "I want to be your father." You have a relationship with me that is meaningful, and I am interested in you."

There are few things that alter a man's life more than becoming a father. Being entrusted with someone else's care and responsibility is a huge responsibility, but nothing is more fulfilling than becoming a father and witnessing your child progressively mature into adulthood, receiving ample return of your devotion, and having their value validated. With any luck, these parenting advice pieces can help dads who are attempting to learn how to be involved, encouraging, and caring fathers.

A father's significance in a child's life

Although anyone can father a child, fatherhood is a lifetime commitment. Every child has a position in their life that no one else can fill: that of their father. A child's development and eventual identity may be greatly influenced by this role.

Fathers and the Development of Emotions

Fathers are essential to a child's emotional development, just like mothers are. Dads are the ones that set and uphold the rules for their children. In addition, they look to their fathers to give them a sense of emotional and physical stability. Youngsters aspire to make their fathers proud, and a supportive father encourages personal development and fortitude. Research indicates that a child's cognitive and social development is significantly impacted by their fathers' affectionate and supporting behavior. Additionally, it fosters a general sense of wellbeing and self-assurance.

Fathers Establish the Standard for Interactions with Others

Fathers shape not just our inner selves but also the relationships we have with others as we mature. What a child searches for in other people is influenced by the way their father raises them. The child's understanding of the significance of the relationship with his or her father will determine who is picked as a friend, lover, and spouse. The manner in which a parent interacts with his children will determine the way in which those youngsters interact with others.

Dads and Their Offspring

Young girls look to their fathers for emotional support and protection. A father demonstrates to his daughter what makes a healthy relationship with a man. When a daughter reaches dating age, she will seek out guys who share her father's affection and gentleness. A powerful and brave parent will find that his children relate well to other men who share his qualities.

Dads and Their Offspring

Boys take their father's character as a model for themselves, while girls base their interactions with others on it. From an early age, boys will look to their fathers for approval. Humans learn how to live in the world by emulating the actions of individuals around them as they grow up. A little kid who grows up with a caring and respectful father would likely grow up in a similar manner. Young boys seek other masculine figures to set the "rules" on how to behave and get by in the world when their father isn't there.

So remember to tell your dad you appreciate him and that you love him today!

I was just telling a friend that the four days I spent with my children were the happiest days of my life. Those were moments of pure, inexplicable bliss for me. And each time I had that newborn in my arms, I can still recall feeling amazed and overpowered by the work at hand.

I was unaware of the numerous additional responsibilities that come with being a father at the time, so I was just thinking about my duty to safeguard and support each new little life. A man's roles increase when he becomes a father. He bears the ultimate responsibility of nurturing another human life in addition to being accountable for himself and his children's mother. He must master the art of donning a wide variety of hats in order to accomplish this.

These are five crucial but sometimes disregarded functions that fathers play.

1. Inspirational

As a father, you are occasionally a friend, a coach, and a helper. Encouraging your kids to be productive and grow healthily each day is one of your responsibilities. I discovered that my children don't always have the self-motivation to develop their character, self-control, and spirituality to the fullest extent possible. I therefore frequently feel compelled to step in and encourage them when I recognize that potential, sometimes in a forceful or imaginative way. This can occasionally be achieved using plans, rewards, timetables, or even just explicit expectations.

2. The Enforcer

The issue of fatherlessness is very important in today's culture. And the lack of the necessary male presence and leadership that many children in fatherless homes experience is one of their biggest disadvantages. Having an enforcer in the house is a big aspect of having a father. Whether they like it or not, children inherently react differently to male authority, particularly inside the home. The fact that dad is the primary upholder of boundaries and family rules at home also greatly eases the burden of raising a woman.

3. Motivator

"All children adore constructive parental guidance."
Being a child's biggest fan and cheerleader is one of the best ways to support them, as children are born with a yearning for their father's attention and praise. It can help a lot to give them regular compliments and encouragement in their areas of strength. When I tell my kids encouraging things like, "You're doing a great job," or "I'm so glad you're mine," I've personally noticed a change in their

behavior. All children like constructive parental guidance.

4. Instructor

Without instruction, your youngster will never pick up certain life lessons and abilities. Teaching our kids to be good life learners is a part of being a father. Your child needs your deliberate involvement in everything from learning to ride a bike to managing positive relationships with people of the opposite sex and everything in between. Yes, it requires some effort and inconvenience, but in the end, it is well worth it.

5. Guidance

Children also face difficulties. Adults sometimes find it easy to overlook this since their issues appear so little. When you were a child, do you recall how little things seemed enormous? Children are not equipped to deal with life's challenges on an instinctive level. That's because they're not grownups yet; they're still children. They frequently require guidance, clarification, and counsel. Dad, make it your mission to be your kids' primary advisor and first choice for guidance. Since they're going to receive it from someone, why not you?

Chapter 2

Honoring Your Father: 8 Ways To Express Your Love And Thanks This Father's Day

It's time to plan a little something extra special for Dad on this Father's Day. Continue reading to discover how to make Father's Day a special day, from spending time together to making unique gifts and surprises.

Celebrated on Father's Day, we pay tribute to the amazing men in our lives who have taken on the role of father figure. It's the ideal chance to thank and show our love for the steadfast support, direction, and affection our fathers have given us.

This year, consider these 8 sincere methods to truly express our gratitude for our fathers, rather than settling for the typical corny gifts. These suggestions will assist you in making enduring memories and transforming Father's Day into a very important and amazing occasion! Continue reading to learn more!

What's the Meaning of Father's Day?

A unique day set aside to honor and celebrate fathers and father figures is Father's Day. It's a day to show them how much we love and appreciate them for their significant contribution to our lives. It is observed on different dates in many nations throughout the world. It stands for the widespread understanding of the value of paternity and the desire to respect and value fathers on a global scale. Father's Day customs and cultural importance might change among cultures and geographical areas.

Father's Day honors fathers for their contributions to their families and the good influence they have on their lives. It honors the special roles fathers play in raising, caring for, and developing their kids as a whole. It emphasizes how vital their love, support, and advice are. It also offers a chance to sincerely thank and show thanks to fathers for their love, devotion, and sacrifices. It's a day to honor their dedication, altruism, and the various ways they improve the lives of their family. It acts as a prompt to value and respect the influence that fathers have in our lives.

This Father's Day, there are eight ways to express your gratitude to your father.

1. Take Time Out for Each Other

Time has become a valuable resource in the fast-paced world of today. Your whole attention is one of the most precious gifts you can give your father. Organize a fun-filled activity or excursion for the two of you, like going fishing, hiking in the mountains, or just having dinner together. You show how much you value your father's company and presence by making time for him. This could even be as simple as scheduling some time to have a deep talk with your father. In this discussion, express your ideas, aspirations, and life experiences. You will gain a deeper understanding of one another and develop an intimate emotional bond through this candid and open discussion.

Father's Day can also be an occasion to commemorate and look back on special memories. Spend some time watching home films, going through old photo albums, or visiting important places from your history. Your bond will strengthen as a result of this sentimental trip, which will also bring back wonderful memories for your father.

When you write in your journal, include pictures and videos, and go over old media with your father.
Journey offers you an ideal platform to preserve your most treasured memories in the form of images, films, and even voice notes! You can add and save media to your Journal entries on Journey, and you can see them whenever you'd like. Look back on your best moments and experiences with your dad on Father's Day by easily adding images, videos, gifs, and music to your journal entries. You may also relive your memories by viewing pictures and videos from a week, a month, or even a year or two ago with Journey's "Throwback" function!

2. Prepare His Favorite Dish for Him.

Making a special lunch for your father is a lovely act of love, and food has a way of uniting people. It might have deep significance in expressing your gratitude. Making your father a special dinner shows that you are a nurturing person who is concerned about his health. It's a loving and considerate gesture that shows how much you want to give him a wonderful and memorable experience. You can show your dad that you respect his unique tastes and preferences by preparing his favorite dinner. It demonstrates that you are aware of his preferences and that you have taken the time to prepare something that is especially catered to his gastronomic needs.

Food has a special power to evoke feelings and build relationships. You can bring back memories of dinner table conversations by cooking your dad's favorite dish. It lets you remember happy times spent sharing delectable meals with loved ones and reminisce about family get-togethers and festivities.

Find his favorite recipe or make a beloved family dish. He will surely feel warmed by the care and attention to detail in the meal, which will bring back fond memories of evenings spent around the dinner table!

3. Make a Customized Gift: Rather than purchasing a store-bought item, think about making a present that is specifically catered to your father's hobbies. A bespoke artwork, a handcrafted photo album filled with priceless memories, or a playlist of his all-time favorite tunes are just a few examples of the unique gifts that show how much you care.

A personalized gift serves as a concrete memento of your love and gratitude for your father. It is heartfelt and will be treasured for many years to come. Your father will be reminded of your thoughtfulness and the unique link you share each time he sees or utilizes the gift. Personalized presents can also be flexible and tailored to your father's requirements or hobbies at any point in his life. You can customize the gift to fit his current interests or hobbies, whether it's an emotional souvenir, personalized accessory, or item relevant to his pastime.

This goes above and beyond the typical thank-you card and shows how much thought, work, and personal connection you have put into it. It turns into a treasured keepsake of your gratitude and love, capturing the special relationship you share with your father.

4. Compose a Customized Letter

Sometimes the most profound effects come from the simplest gestures. Spend some time writing a sincere letter to your father, detailing your feelings and views. Tell him about special times in your life, memories you have of him, and how he has influenced it. Your father would cherish a handwritten, personal letter as a memento for years to come.

Writing a handwritten letter gives you a personal and meaningful approach to communicate your feelings. It gives you a chance to express how much you appreciate, love, and thank your father. Written words leave a lasting impression and have the power to convey feelings that spoken words may not always be able to. You must also consider how your father has influenced your life. It enables you to take a time to reflect on the knowledge gained, the assistance obtained, and the experiences shared. You can acknowledge and value the influence your father has had on the development of your moral compass and sense of self through this introspection.

Think back for a while on the things your dad has done for you and the meaning she holds in your life. Tell her how grateful you are and how much you adore him. To keep him motivated and pleased, you might even insert little messages of encouragement and positive affirmations in your letter. This would be ideal if words of affirmation are her love language! Your father will treasure this small act of kindness for years to come. It can mean the world to him.

5. Arrange an Unexpected Visit.

A lovely method to let your father know how much you care is to give him surprises. Plan a surprise excursion or activity that fits his interests. It may be a weekend getaway, concert tickets, or even sports event tickets.

Father's Day is made more exciting and joyful by surprise outings. It takes your father by surprise, which makes the party more joyous and exciting. The element of surprise shows how much care and effort you put into organizing a unique experience just for him.

It's important to carefully examine your father's interests, hobbies, or preferences while organizing a surprise outing. It demonstrates that you have gotten to know him well and have taken the effort to choose an activity that suits his interests. It is clear from your careful thought process that you much value his uniqueness.

6. Discuss a Father-Son or Father-Daughter Activity.

Take part in something that can strengthen your relationship and help you and your father make new memories. Engaging in a common activity, such as cooking classes, biking rides, or golfing, will strengthen your relationship and open up new avenues for meaningful communication.

Engaging in a task alongside your father offers a chance for education and development. Learning a new skill, taking up a new hobby, or spending time together doing something you both enjoy provides for the sharing of information, wisdom, and important life lessons. This mutual education fortifies the relationship and fosters a sense of unity.

Partaking in an activity with your father-son or father-daughter creates opportunities for deep talks. It fosters a laid-back and friendly atmosphere where you can converse freely, exchange ideas, and get to know one another better. This dialogue builds a supportive friendship and fortifies the emotional bond. Reconciling around a particular pastime that is deeply ingrained in your family's customs or history strengthens the link between generations. It enables you to commemorate common beliefs, traditions, or rites while transferring sentimental customs from your father to next generations. Family bonds are strengthened by this feeling of continuity and respect for ancestral customs.

7. Give thanks on social media.

Social media platforms provide a large audience in the digital era for you to express your gratitude for your father. Write a sincere post that conveys your love and gratitude and includes a treasured photo. Sharing your thankfulness on social media makes a digital record that you can look back on at a later time. It turns into a material symbol of your love and gratitude for your father. You and your dad can revisit the post, relive the feelings, and treasure the public proclamation of your relationship. It's an open expression of gratitude that will surely fill your father with pride and make him feel loved.

Expressing your appreciation for your father on social media gives you a chance to publicly thank him for his love, support, and influence on your life. It enables you to publicly thank your father for his role as a father, allowing friends, family, and even his acquaintances to see and participate in the celebration.

8. Encourage His Interests and Hobbies.

Engage in conversation about your father's interests and passions. Take part in a pastime he loves, go to his favorite sporting events, or assist him with a do-it-yourself project. You become an active part of your father's world by taking part in his interests and pastimes. It demonstrates that you respect his interests and are open to participating with him in enjoyable activities. Your enthusiastic participation shows how much you value his hobbies and the work he puts into them.

Spending time with your father and connecting over his interests and pastimes is a great opportunity. It fosters a shared experience where you may laugh, connect, and have deep talks. Your bond is strengthened and a deeper connection based on shared interests is fostered by this time spent together. You can learn more about your father as a person by immersing yourself in his interests and pastimes. It lets you appreciate the things that make him happy and see the world from his point of view. This comprehension enhances empathy and fortifies your emotional bond.

On Father's Day, we commemorate and appreciate the fathers in our lives who have contributed greatly to our lives. We can show our fathers how much we appreciate and adore them by embracing sincere gestures instead of standard gifts. These eight suggestions provide an assortment of methods to turn Father's Day into an unforgettable event, ranging from spending time together to making unique gifts and surprises. To genuinely make this day unique for your father, never forget that the best gift you can give him is the warmth and sincerity of your love and gratitude.

Greetings on Father's Day!

Chapter 3

The Father's Place in the Family: Both Historically and Presently.

Dads now have more responsibilities, and involvement is essential.
A child's mental and physical health are greatly impacted by the role that a father plays in the home. A child's psychological well-being and lifetime relationships are positively correlated when they have a positive relationship with a father figure. We examine the father role and its evolution in the last few years.

A Father's Place in the Family

In a household, father figures can take on a variety of roles. Remember that the term "father" refers to more than only husband and wife connections or merely biological links.

Just as significant parent-child interactions are provided by same-sex couples, transgender males who are parents, and single fathers as they are by families headed by a husband and wife. A child who grows up in a particular kind of home does not necessarily have the best father-child bond.

Fatherly figures:

They could be stepparents or not biologically related to the child or children they look after.
perhaps adopted a kid or kids
They might not have legal responsibility for the kids they look after.
The quality of the parent-child relationship is the most crucial component, regardless of the structure of the family.

The Godfather's Role

What Does a Father Do in Today's Families?
In contrast to earlier times, a growing number of men nowadays take an equal role in both caring for their families and raising their

children. This strengthens the spousal bond while also providing a good model for the kids.

In fact, even when their baby was fussy, a study of married couples who had recently given birth to their first child revealed that when a father contributed to these activities, there was an overall decrease in annoyance for both partners. Fathers can play a variety of roles in the family, such as:

Contributors with money
dependable companions
devoted parents
parents who stay at home
Healthy co-parenting even with a separation or divorce

Why Having a Father Is Vital

A father figure has a big impact on a child's life and wellness. The father is one of the child's first role models and interactions in families where the father figure is present. Children absorb relational experiences and are incredibly perceptive and sensitive creatures.

These formative exchanges with their father influence both the father-daughter and the father-son relationships by acting as a model for what constitutes a healthy connection. This implies that unhealthful father figure connections can have a substantial negative influence on a child's psychological health as well as their unconscious relationship decisions as adults.

When a child and father get along well, the youngster will likely grow up to be more confident and self-assured adults and form more enduring connections with other men.
A child who has psychological anguish and finds it difficult to build good relationships as an adult may have a bad relationship with their father.
Remember that the internalized relational template that develops in early childhood is extremely hard to change. Although this foundation can be altered, doing so frequently requires highly developed awareness in addition to substantial psychotherapy interventions to transform these ingrained, frequently unconscious brain pathways.

The Changing Nature of the Father in Modern Society

The concept of the "involved father" has just been recognizable in the last several decades. Dads have been actively involved in parenting more recently, despite the fact that previously, men's identities were strongly linked to their occupations.

Of the 7% of men who reported being stay-at-home dads, 24% said that their main motivation was to care for their child or children.

Men felt pressured to be involved fathers in 49% of cases.

49% of adults said they thought men were under more pressure to go back to work after having a kid.

How the Pandemic Has Positively Impacted Fatherhood

We were all compelled to seek shelter in our houses when the pandemic struck in 2020 while medical professionals figured out how to address this medical emergency. Fathers had the rare chance to work from home and spend more time with their children during this period of isolation.

Investigators have discovered that "almost 70% of fathers across race, class, educational attainment, and political affiliation in the United States closer to their children during the coronavirus pandemic." Additionally, the research revealed that since the pandemic began, over half of American fathers:

Give their kids greater appreciation
are more sensitive to the emotions of their kids
Increase their level of involvement in their kids' everyday activities and conversations.
Surprisingly, a study conducted in October 2020 revealed that 46% of fathers believed they were spending the appropriate amount of time with their children, compared to only 36% in 2017. Furthermore, the proportion of fathers who feel they spend insufficient time with their children has decreased by 15% (from 63% in 2017).

How the Pandemic Affected Fathers' Perspectives on Work

More flexible work arrangements were another benefit of the pandemic. Many dads now see their former duties differently, even if most firms have returned to their pre-crisis state.

Only 26% of fathers planned to resume their pre-pandemic work, but many of them desired to seek less demanding positions. 25% of fathers wanted to cut back on the number of hours they work.
Rethinking fathers' job goals and the importance of striking a work-life balance is a significant step in assisting families in preserving strong bonds.

Must Be Aware

The pandemic altered the way that many businesses run. This is helpful for both new and seasoned fathers who want to be more engaged in their children's lives, so take the time to look into options that will provide you with the balance you need to create a better life for your family and yourself.

Important Duties a Father Should Have

When it comes to good parenting, a father's responsibilities could be:

- Exemplifying positive interpersonal conduct with other adults and your other caregiver, if applicable exhibiting kindness, loving, and unhindered time spent bonding with your child.

- Using healthy methods to show affection. Taking good care of your physical and mental health and setting an example of appropriate behavior when assistance is required.

- Being tolerant and merciful. Avoid forcing or projecting your beliefs upon your offspring.

- Allowing your child to take the initiative in some circumstances and giving them the freedom to be who they are extending empathy and acceptance.

- Instructing and demonstrating suitable dispute resolution techniques as well as good communication techniques.

- Having healthy boundaries and using proper discipline (no screaming, violence, spanking, withholding of affection, or extended punishment)

What Function Do the Mother and Father Serve in a Family?

Remember that father figures might be active in families other than those headed by a mother and father; in today's world, parents typically share childrearing duties.

Different Parental Roles Depending on the Family
Regarding particular duties, these will differ substantially based on the requirements of every

distinct household. But in happy families, it's ideal for both parents to be adaptable and able to fill the same tasks, all the while supporting one another in their roles as spouses and parents. It's acceptable for the roles that parents play in today's homes to differ greatly from one another. No family has to behave in the same way as another.

What Are Parents' Responsibilities?

Mothers and fathers may divide home duties equally or devise a mutually beneficial arrangement based on the dynamics inside the family. In terms of parenting, it is ideal for both the mother and the father to have positive relationships with their child or children and to share equal parental responsibilities.

The Value of a Parent

A father's influence on a child's development and promotion of both physical and mental well-being is substantial. The most crucial element of the parent-child relationship is the quality of the connection, not the fact that the child and father are blood relatives, regardless of how the father figure is related to the child or what nickname the child uses for this parent. Therefore, being a positive presence is the most vital function of a father.

What Are A Father's Three Main Responsibilities?

Fathers have traditionally played three main functions in practically every culture that has been studied: provider, disciplinarian, and protector. Before we get into each of these responsibilities, it's crucial to recognize that mothers play just as big of a role in these three roles as fathers do in many two-parent households nowadays. Mothers safeguard their children by fastening their seatbelts, placing them in car seats, keeping an eye on their computer usage, and scanning their surroundings for any potential threats. Just like fathers, mothers labor outside the home to support their families. In addition, women now tend to be more strict with their kids than they were in the past, when we would hear things like "You wait until your father gets home."

Although we are talking about the significance of the father figure in a child's life for the purposes of this course, moms also play vital roles in their children's lives.

<u>Defender.</u> When a female is expecting, one of the tactics we've employed is to encourage men to baby- or child-proof their home. What actions may they take to get the house ready for the child? Men can shield their kids from threats within the home by doing this, for example. They are also capable of shielding their kids from outside threats. This is particularly crucial in areas with greater rates of violence since there's a chance the child will be exposed to criminal activities or gang involvement.

Mothers often view the world through the lens of their children. Fathers frequently view their kids in the context of the wider world. The typical focus of moms is on shielding their children from external threats like bullies, strangers, nasty pets, accidents, and illness. She wishes for her child to never experience this. Dads' paternal instinct also aims to keep unpleasant things from happening, but in the event that they do, they want to take the necessary steps to equip their child to handle these kinds of risks. Dads frequently make an effort to get their kids ready for situations when they may encounter outside threats like hostile strangers, vicious dogs, lightning, bullies, falls, or mishaps. For the child, both of these roles are significant. Dad is getting the kid ready, and mom is watching out for him.

Fathers also perform the role of guardian by keeping an eye on their children's social surroundings and getting to know their friends and peers. Do we also know what's in the house when our kids visit another family? Are there any guns in their house? Is the neighborhood safe? What steps should I take to keep my child safe from potentially dangerous situations? By establishing their surroundings, fathers also ensure the protection of their children. Stated differently, they have the ability to observe their environment (home, neighborhood, community, etc.) and promote safe choices while also removing potential hazards from the child's path.

Supplier. A father's capacity to support his family is a function of his manhood, sense of obligation, and sense of identity. The teachings about what it means to be a male, a spouse, and a father vary among cultures. One of the main responsibilities that fathers play in many of those societies is that of a provider. It is said that "real men bring home the bacon," provide for their families, work in factories, mines, and forests, or tend to the fields. As the family's provider, they must accept the risks associated with their jobs. As I indicated, fathers are no longer the only breadwinners in many two-parent households nowadays, but they still play a crucial role in their families.

Disciplinary. Fathers generally have high expectations when it comes to their child's future preparation. They want their child to be successful, to see the future, and to have high expectations for themselves. Fathers must therefore be present to educate their children how to control their urges, how to remain composed under pressure, and how to handle circumstances in which they do not pose a threat to themselves or others. Many fathers are playing the role of the disciplinarian in the American society that is currently in vogue, but they must do so in a way that is courteous and safe. It cannot be done in a violent manner since males who grow up in violent homes often carry that trait through to their own families. It's crucial for the father to use his physical presence in this capacity of disciplinarian to teach his child how to react appropriately to various situations.

Chapter 4

Importance of Fathers

Dads are unquestionably significant. They are so crucial that a poor one has the power to send their youngster into a tailspin. A good father can help their children grow into successful, happy, balanced individuals by providing them with emotional, physical, financial, and spiritual support. If you have ever lost a father, either by death or abandonment, you understand the importance of fathers.

Loving their child's mother is one of the best and most crucial things a man can do. This sets an example for the men their daughters will one day marry and demonstrates to sons what a good man should be like.

Although it may seem simplistic and outdated, all of this is real.

A father who is good is worth their weight in gold.

Fathers' Crucial Contribution to Their Children's Emotional Development

Fathers are important. Just like kids need moms to love them, show interest in them, and attend to their needs, children also need fathers to make them feel important and understood.

Fathers—and father figures—have a significant impact on the growth of their offspring. While women give their children distinct things, males have something as vital to provide their offspring. The distinctions between males and females in parenting are not predetermined; rather, each family must learn these distinctions for itself.

Fathers are significant because their partners value them as well. Children learn how to relate from their parents, thus how well or poorly their parents handle their own relationships will have a significant impact on how well or poorly they do in the future. This is not to suggest that parents must always be flawless. However, it is crucial that kids witness their parents cooperating to try to resolve the issues that occasionally arise in every household.
Being a father is a big step for any man. No one truly knows what it will be like for them until it actually happens. There are many various ways

to respond, of course, and this pamphlet does not try to prescribe how a father should behave. The most crucial things are to be interested in your kids, have fun with them, and trust your gut. The key takeaway is:

Whether and how men participate can have a significant impact on their children's life; if they choose not to participate, both fathers and children will lose out on the chance to have a fulfilling and joyful connection.

To Getting Ready To Be A Father

Men should be fully involved in the planning process for the birth of a child because they too have a lot to learn about adjusting to their new position. The amount of time fathers spend getting ready for parenthood might have a significant impact on their level of involvement once the baby is born. If you plan to become an adoptive father, getting ready for the baby's arrival on both an emotional and physical level is equally crucial.

It's possible to view childrearing and raising children as a woman's domain, and males may occasionally feel as though they don't truly belong. Men may experience intense jealousy towards their pregnant partner without even realizing it. In response, they can start working on a lot of new initiatives for themselves.

For the father's bond with both their partner and the child, being present for the delivery can be quite beneficial. The thought of attending prenatal lessons might make men uncomfortable or even ashamed. But if fathers are ready for the experience, it will be less traumatic for them both physically and emotionally during the birth.

Fathers may find it difficult to participate as much as they would want because the health system does not always suit their demands. For example, prenatal lessons might take place during the day, and employers might not be understanding.

Which Sort of Dad Are You Going to Be?

A multitude of experiences shape the behavior of fathers. Our upbringing greatly shapes the men and women we become as parents. This is deeply ingrained. Frequently, we could not fully understand the reasons behind our actions or reactions. For example, men who were never allowed to feel furious with their own parents could find it extremely difficult to deal with their child's rage.

It is possible for new fathers to put in excessive hours at work without realizing that they are using it as a shield from domestic difficulties. They might eventually regret doing this.
How well a child and their parents get along is one of the most essential things in the world. It is a sad reality that many families break up when their children are young.
Establishing a joyful environment at home is the best start that parents can give their kids. Parents should work together to resolve conflicts and come to agreements on how to do this. This holds true for a variety of situations, including taking care of the infant, changing diapers, and sharing the parents' bed.

Young newborns in particular are highly perceptive to the emotional climate in their environment. Children will react if there is tension between the parents, whether it be related to their relationship or other issues like money worries.

We occasionally require assistance from someone else if it is difficult for us to comprehend or manage with what is happening. This might manifest itself directly or indirectly, such as in the form of tantrums, sleep issues, or other behavioral issues. The Child Psychotherapy Trust's pamphlets aid parents in comprehending their evolving relationship with their growing children.

The Early Years

Typically, fathers misjudge the amount of change a newborn will bring about in their home. Some guys might attempt to act as though nothing has changed at all. However, most parents discover that they have less money, less sex, and less sleep after having a child!

It could take some time before you feel deeply connected to your child.

After the baby is delivered, fathers should strive to take some time off from work to be with their growing family.

Though it is frequently overlooked, it has lately come to light that males can experience postpartum depression in addition to moms. In fact, a new baby's birth may sometimes be much more taxing on a father than it is on a mother. Everyone anticipates that the new mother would be preoccupied with the infant, but if the father is not actively participating in the baby's care, he could feel redundant and useless. This may be particularly challenging if the father believes he cannot fulfill the usual role of being the earner since he is also unemployed.

If you are struggling to adjust to the new environment, it is crucial that you talk to someone. Dads might be able to express their feelings to their spouse, but talking to someone outside the family might be simpler. A friend or family member who is also a parent may be able to offer support, as might the doctor or health visitor.

Taking Care of the Infant

It makes no difference how a parent chooses to interact with his kids; what matters is that he engages with them.

While some men barely give their babies any attention at all, others may put in so much effort to be excellent dads that they begin to compete with mothers to see who can be the best at raising their children. They could become so interested in housework and infant care that the mother begins to feel a little pushed out.

Fathers should make an effort to strike a balance so that they can support and assist their mothers without taking charge or undermining her. Nobody says this is a simple task, especially because you and your spouse are probably feeling especially sensitive and worn out right now.

Dads and Their Companions

Fathers play a crucial role in relationships, not only for themselves and their partner but also for the sake of the children. In the family, it really doesn't matter who does what. For example, while deciding what each partner should do around the house, it is most important for parents to come to a decision that pleases them both.

Couples can only accomplish this if they both recognize the value of their personal relationship with one another. In order to maintain their attempt at maintaining a distinct relationship as a couple, fathers have a significant role to perform. It's incredibly simple to overlook this because you're too excited about the new baby and your newfound parenthood.

Children will gain a great deal by realizing that their parents are independent adults, and their perception of their parents' connection is crucial.

Fathers must so ensure that they maintain communication with their partners. Talking about feelings is one of the most frequent grievances women have about their spouses. This may reveal a lot about the way we raise young boys, and it can be difficult to alter, but it is crucial that we make an effort. In this manner, the likelihood that a couple can resolve issues as they come up is significantly increased.

Dads and Their Offspring

There is no one "correct" method for guys to interact with infants and kids. Compassionate expressions are as vital as playful ones. What counts are the father's happiness and his desire to build a bond with his child.

When it comes to their children, fathers and mothers frequently act very differently:

They might engage in tougher, tumble games.

Their newborns notice that their parents speak differently to them and react accordingly by changing the way they move.

Researchers can determine who is speaking to a newborn even when they are unable to see them by observing how they react. This is an alternative form of care that is beneficial for babies.

Fathers have a crucial influence in the lives of both boys and girls. Having a close relationship with both parents is beneficial for children, as one provides them with something different from the other. A father's position is still crucial as his children get older, but it evolves.

Boys: Your father could serve as an inspiration. Boys' sociability may be greatly influenced by their father, according to some research.
Girls: Especially in their teenage years, having a positive relationship with their father can have a significant impact on their sense of identity and self-worth.
Teens: During the adolescent years, fathers are particularly significant. They might assist in establishing boundaries or have a specific function in assisting the teenagers in becoming more independent.

Fathers Alone or Fathers Who Are Not Together

It is extremely terrible for all parties involved to be separated from their children, but there are ways to make it work for both of you.

It is important to remember that both of you are still parents, and children are typically loyal to both parents despite what either parent may think. You and your ex-partner still need to work together as parents, if not as a couple. It will help if you can maintain good terms with the children's mother, even though this may be difficult. In this way, even though you are living apart, the kids will see you cooperating for their best interests.

It is very simple for unrelated problems to skew the image and impair your judgment. Outside assistance, such as from friends, coworkers, or organizations, can help you concentrate on your kids' needs.

It might be challenging to stay in regular contact with your children for a variety of various practical and emotional reasons. Seeing your kids solely on the weekends or on special occasions can feel quite fake compared to the informal daily interactions you have from sharing a home. You could become disconnected from their hobbies. Even when their parents are still living together, at various ages, the last thing kids want is to be seen out with them. However, you continue to play a crucial role in their life, and they depend on you to support them, therefore handling this in any way is very vital. Maintaining communication, whether by phone conversations, emails, or postcards, is beneficial.

Fathers Who Are Alone

Even for two parents, raising a child may be difficult, let alone one. Being a single parent is a difficult job, and it can be taxing to shoulder all of the duty by yourself. A great deal will rely on the circumstances surrounding this.

If the mother of the children has moved out, you will all need to deal with intensely hurtful and perplexed emotions about how she could have done so. If you are experiencing similar thoughts, it could be quite difficult to discover a sincere manner to support the kids in this area.

It can be simpler to support them in maintaining a positive internal image of their mother if she has passed away. They will continue to feel irrationally about what has transpired even then. If you want to support someone when you are also grieving, you must have tolerance. Fathers must learn to feel maternal inside themselves when the mother of their children passes away.

All single parents deal with a lot of personal and practical challenges; men confront even more as it is so uncommon for them to be the only parent.

Typically, loneliness is a major problem.

Employers might not be as understanding.

When they are in primary school, mothers organize a large portion of their social lives. As a father, it might be harder, but not impossible, to be a part of this circle.

Compared to mothering, fathering is frequently a more private affair. It is possible that single fathers will have a tougher time getting the assistance they need because males don't communicate to each other about parenting in the same way that women do.

Various Types of Families

Fathers in Step

Even though stepmothers are typically portrayed negatively in children's literature, adopting the role of father to children who are not your own is incredibly challenging. Stepfathers may worry about this and find it difficult to feel "fatherly." It is crucial, therefore, to consider the child's feelings and act in a considerate and suitable manner.

Naturally, a lot depends on the specifics. Whether or not he is truly present very often, or at all, many kids do have another father. If the child's biological father has passed away, feelings are probably considerably stronger.

It should come as no surprise that kids could use this as a weapon in family disputes when they're under stress. Respecting the children's feelings toward their biological father is crucial, as is keeping in mind how difficult this must be for them—if their father truly loves them, then why has he abandoned them? It's possible that despite the child's cognitive justifications for their father's absence, the experience of being abandoned remains relatively unaffected. This can negatively impact the child's sense of self. They might even try to put the blame on their new stepfather for displacing their "real" father. The children could feel conflicted about their biological father's new spouse, and they might feel competitive with their new stepbrothers and sisters.

A child's relationship with their birth father could be tense.

As you can see, assuming the position of a stepfather is quite challenging. Handling it well requires a great deal of subtlety, and you won't always be able to do it correctly—if only because the kids might need an excuse.

However, just like with biological parents, the most important thing is how successfully the two individuals who are now the "parental couple" work things out together. The kids must understand that although their stepfather cannot take the place of their biological father, he does play a fatherly role in this new family. To assist her children in accepting this, he will require his partner's assistance.

Naturally, these issues don't always come up. Stepdads can infuse family dynamics with a new energy, easing tensions and opening doors to creative problem-solving.

Fathers Who Adopt

To become a father, adoptive fathers had to go through a rigorous and occasionally taxing process. This requires a great lot of introspection and the willingness to face personal concerns that other fathers would never have to. This presents a challenge for some men, who believe they must prove themselves in a manner that their biological fathers would not. However, because he is very conscious of his desire to be a parent and the decision he has taken, it can also deepen the bond between a father and his adopted kid.

As kids get older, they could have difficult-to-answer queries concerning their biological parents. They might be interested in learning more about their birth families and have a curiosity about them. They might be interested in meeting them in order to learn more about their own perspective on the events surrounding their birth.

Thinking of the child's interest about their genetic origins as completely natural can help fathers withstand feelings of rejection and hostility that may be painful and difficult to explain. Sometimes, when they are upset or furious, they may lash out at their adopted fathers.

Fathers in Foster Care

Foster fathers are apt to encounter intricate obstacles as well. A kid may have entered foster care due to a variety of reasons, such as brief family troubles or severe parental issues, such as physical or sexual abuse. It's possible that the foster child enters your household with a negative perception of what fathers can do for them.

Speak with the child's social worker to obtain as much information as you can about their experiences. It is imperative and beneficial. It will be simpler to ignore their mistrust, antagonism, rejection, or even seductiveness if you have some notion of how they have felt about males. This can assist you in putting up with the really challenging behavior you'll probably have to deal with.

Finding sensitive ways to discuss your foster child's feelings with you may also be made easier by your understanding. You might get assistance with this sensitive duty from your support worker, the children's social worker, or a member of your local Child and Adolescent Mental Health Team.

Fathers of the same sex

Gay couples who decide to become parents may become foster parents or adoptive fathers, who may or may not be the biological father. It's important to keep in mind that males in all these diverse types of families might encounter some difficult obstacles, some of which are exclusive to homosexual fathers.

It's quite normal for a child to have questions about their origins, especially concerns about the mother who conceived and gave birth to them. It might be helpful to give simple, kid-friendly responses for these inquiries.

It can also be crucial to find channels for discussing any worries you may have about having two dads and no mother.

It is vital to consider what your child is conveying as well as the various sensitivities that parents have. Different worries may surface at different stages of your child's development, especially between fathers and their teenage daughters when mom is not there. You may also be concerned that your child will face discrimination for having fathers of the same sex or that you will be singled out.

Look into any parent organizations in your area as they may be a great resource for help.

<u>Practical Advice For Fathers</u>

A good parent spends a disproportionate amount of time with his children, compared to the impact he has on them. Although there is no set way to be a good father, studies have shown that when a father supports and is devoted to his children, it makes a big difference in their lives.

Seize the chance to participate in prenatal or parenting classes as an expectant father. Being mentally and physically prepared will benefit both you and your child.

Fathers of newborns frequently feel jealous, excluded, and like they're "having their nose put out of joint." Sometimes the causes are clear: fathers who feel incapable of caring for a small child are either kept out of their child's life or excluded themselves. However, the causes aren't always clear-cut and can have anything to do with the father's past. Try talking to your partner or someone else about the problems you're having.

Even though it can be challenging to stay in touch as a divorced father, your child will truly gain from your constant interest in them.

Prove to your child that even though you are living somewhere else, they are still very much on your mind. Recall noteworthy events, including birthdays.

Take up any assistance that is offered to you as a single father. You and your child will not benefit from continuing to battle on your own.

Although stepfathers are frequently given a poor rap, you can positively impact your stepchildren's life by being considerate and sensitive.

Chapter 5

The Dad-to-Be Guide: 10 Action Items to Take Before Becoming a Father

1. Acquire the fundamentals

There are a lot of tactical things to know when getting ready to become a father. We are discussing practical knowledge that recently became parents should possess. To begin with, you need make sure you understand some fundamental infant abilities. You should become familiar with several everyday baby skills, such as how to:

Hug your child.
A diaper change.
Create a stronger bond with your infant by doing "kangaroo care."
Give your child a burp.
Wrap your infant in a swaddle.
Put in a car seat.
Give your infant a safe bath.

Calm your finicky child.
Prepare formula or store human milk for breastfeeding.
Make your area babyproof.
Adhere to baby safe sleeping practices.
Apply basic first aid to infants and children.

Books and internet resources abound that cover all of these topics and more. consulting community resources or healthcare facilities in your area. They frequently hold classes for new parents where you may learn all the ins and outs of keeping your kid happy, healthy, fed, and safe. To gain guidance on getting ready for a new role in their families, they might also provide programs designed especially for new fathers.

2. Select infant equipment
Without a doubt, bringing a baby into the house means bringing in some additional furniture. You don't need everything, and it might be overpowering.

diapers? Indeed. Warmer diaper wipes? Call you. bumpers for cribs? Strongly no.

Working together and discussing what you and your spouse need. Choosing what to purchase or add to a baby registry involves more than just joint shopping. The decision you make reveals a lot about your shared parenting style. Additionally, it may spark some crucial discussions.

3. Tidy and arrange

That brand-new baby things needs to go somewhere. If your partner is all about nesting but shouldn't be performing the hard lifting, new dads can assist in getting the house ready for their new baby.

Expectant fathers can get ready for their child by:

Thoroughly cleaning the house so that when your baby arrives, nobody will have to worry about it.

preparing some meals in advance will save you from having to think about cooking from scratch for a while.

Assembling new furniture.

ensuring that the baby's garments are cleaned and stored.

putting up one (or, if your house is two stories high, two) diaper changing stations. For every new diaper, climbing and descending stairs might be quite tiresome.)

4. Arrange the labor division.
Discussing your obligations to your child, your co-parent, and your home will be beneficial if you and your partner are co-residents. These can be especially significant discussions.

You and your partner can reach a mutual understanding on how different home needs will be met by talking about the role you expect to play and understanding each other's needs.

"Some of the tasks they may be used to doing can go undone if your partner is busy, exhausted, or has any limits from their doctor about what they should and shouldn't be doing. This is an opportunity to take up the slack.

After having a child, some spouses who previously had a stable balance of home tasks may need to adjust. You'll also be given some additional, baby-specific duties to complete.

Who will be needing to be fed and changed in the middle of the night? Is it possible to switch roles?

Who's in charge of laundry?

Who is going to cook?

Who will clean the bathroom and how often?

"Perhaps you could agree that you'll start vacuuming and that the dishes don't have to be done at night," he offers. "Any agreement you have works as long as both of you are on board."

5. Take care of your work-life harmony.
You should also make plans for how to handle your professional life. Scheduling is a major aspect of life for any working parent. If possible, you could find that you would benefit from making some changes to your work-life balance as you get ready to become a father.

It's a good idea to plan your time off from work and see if your work obligations can change after your baby is born before the actual birth.

Find out if non-birthing parents are eligible for parental leave at your place of employment.

Some (who may or may not be compensated for it) do. Dads-to-be should make any necessary plans to take time off when their baby arrives and should be aware of any parental benefits or vacation time that their employers may offer before the baby is born.

To make the most of your time at home, you can also think about seeing whether you might benefit from remote work or flexible hours.

6. Arrange for daycare.
Naturally, expecting parents must arrange for who will watch the infant during the day because babies require constant supervision.

Which parent will remain at home?
What qualities are you seeking in a daycare facility or in childcare?
Will a friend or relative help look after your child while you're at work?
Researching potential daycare providers is a crucial aspect of getting ready to become a parent. It's important to keep in mind that many daycare facilities have waiting lists, so if that's the path you choose, you should begin the

process of reducing your options and scheduling visits as soon as possible.

Establish a plan for who will drop off and pick up the infant if they will be away from home while their parents are at work.

7. Organize your financial affairs

The cost of raising children is not surprising. The U.S. Department of Agriculture calculated in 2015 that raising a child costs about $13,000 annually. It's more like $17,000 when converted to 2022 money, according to the Brookings Institution.

Taking into account how your spending plan will handle a new family member as you are ready to become a parent will assist make sure your family stays financially stable. Among the more significant costs in the initial years may be:

baby supplies, such as cots, car seats, and clothing.
childcare.
Daily essentials, such as wipes and diapers (and formula, if applicable).

health coverage.
Costs associated with giving birth in a hospital.

8. Recognize your role during childbirth

Alright, so we are aware that you will not be experiencing the physical strain of labor and delivery. However, you continue to play a significant role in the birth and have a lot of labor support duties ahead of you.

Your job throughout labor and delivery is to assist the birthing parent in every way you can. Thus, discuss with them how you may help.

Being an advocate, being aware of your partner's preferences throughout the birth, and providing any assistance you can are three important ways you may assist with the birth.

Sometimes, that could imply:

taking childbirth education programs to prepare yourself.
when the time comes, getting your partner securely to a birthing center.

offering labor assistance in the form of cold compresses, massages, ice chips, breath coaching, words of encouragement, or other necessities.

Notifying friends and family about announcements and updates.

coordinating (or discouraging) hospital visits.

9. Look after yourself

Making plans for how you'll continue to look after your physical, mental, and social well-being is just as important as thinking about how your life will change once you have a child. Being a healthy person is essential to being a successful parent. We can only offer others a drink when our own cup is full.

It's crucial, but our culture doesn't always support fathers being open and honest about their vulnerabilities or taking time for their personal wellbeing.

Giving up on yourself is not a requirement of being a good parent. It's about knowing how to take care of yourself and balance the demands of other people. Finding that balance is not going to be simple all the time.

Look for strategies to continue taking care of your physical and mental health while you get ready to become a father. Taking care of oneself entails taking care of your child.

"I frequently talk with new dads about making sure they understand that when tensions get too high, it's OK to walk away and to compose yourself after making sure the baby is in a safe place. When we get overwhelmed, it becomes easier to lose our cool."

This is particularly crucial because male caregivers are frequently the ones responsible for occurrences of shaken baby syndrome.

Depending on the individual, taking care of oneself might mean numerous things. It might seem as follows:

getting in sufficient exercise.
eating a diet that is beneficial to your health.
assessing your state of mind.
scheduling downtime for rest and self-care.
savoring the company of your friends and partner.

10. Consider the wider picture

Everything changes when you have a new child in your life. It simply does. It modifies the responsibilities and expectations put on each family member. It's possible that your priorities will shift. The amount of time you allocate to various interests could vary. Your connections might evolve. It's alright. It makes sense.

According to a writer, you have the chance to think about the kind of father you want to be and how your parenting style will reflect that as you reflect on this next chapter in your life.

We tend to parent in a way that is at least somewhat reminiscent of our upbringing, he continues. This is a good opportunity to consider the presumptions you have made based on your personal interactions with your own parents.

"You have this enormous potential there in front of you. Take some time to reflect on the qualities of your own parents that you valued and the qualities that you didn't, and then make some changes.

Think about the following while deciding what kind of parent you want to be:

How am I going to handle matters of discipline?
How will I instill a sense of disappointment in my children?
How am I going to handle the pressures of becoming a parent?
What lifelong teachings am I going to impart to my kid?
It's not necessary for you to know the answers to these huge questions right now. However, figuring out what kind of parent you'll be for your newborn will help establish expectations. It will provide you with a road map for handling anything from helping your adolescent grow up to be a happy, healthy adult to what to do when your toddler bites a friend (it happens!).

Thus, never stop asking inquiries. Continue conversing with your companion. Continue picking up tips from others and expanding your repertoire of new-dad expertise. Perhaps in the not too distant future, you will impart all that you have discovered to others.

"I'm always thrilled to hear from new fathers who want to be prepared rather than going in blind," a writer adds. "No new parent can be prepared for what's ahead, but the more you learn and converse with others, the more assured you can be that you'll be a fantastic father."

Dad, you got this.

Conclusion

Although it can be quite difficult at times, being a father is one of the greatest pleasures and most fulfilling tasks in life. To further address the topic of honesty, being a good father is an extremely difficult task.

Dads had it easier in many ways since they just went about their lives, occasionally attended to their children, and called it a day. We grew up, put our life in motion, and wished for success. No endless self-reflection or yearning for what may have been.

But the good things of being and being a father benefit not just us, our kids, and our family; more importantly, though, they have a big long-term positive impact on everyone in our immediate vicinity.

It's critical for fathers to be involved and present in their families' lives. Set a good example by acting with honesty, integrity, and accountability. Effectively communicate by paying attention to and affirming the emotions of your family. Be kind and loving, and use both words and deeds to let your family know how much you value them. Recognize that being a father can provide difficulties at times, and exercise patience and understanding. Encourage and support your family's ambitions while instilling virtues like kindness, empathy, and respect. Remember to look after your own physical, mental, and emotional well-being in addition to maintaining your relationship with your partner. Ask for help if you need it, please. You can create a solid, loving relationship with your family and community by adhering to these values.

Fathers play a crucial part in families; let's support and uplift them in this capacity. Let's dispel negative gender stereotypes and elevate positive male role models. By encouraging a feeling of camaraderie among men and families, we can help make the world a better place for everyone by offering resources and assistance when required.

In order to create lifelong memories and share experiences with your family, it is crucial for fathers to be actively involved in their daily lives. Set a good example for your family by acting with honesty, integrity, and responsibility. Also, demonstrate to them that perseverance and hard work are necessary to reach objectives. Establish a safe and encouraging environment where your family feels comfortable confiding in you with their ideas and worries. Communicate effectively, listening to and acknowledging their sentiments.

Be kind and loving to your family, letting them know how much you value their accomplishments and milestones in both words and deeds. Being a parent can be difficult at times, so have patience and understanding, and don't be afraid to ask for assistance when you need it. Encourage and support your family's ambitions while instilling virtues like kindness, empathy, and respect.

Remember to look after your own physical, mental, and emotional well-being; make self-care a priority and get help when you need it.

Recognize that a solid and loving connection is the cornerstone of a happy and healthy family, and nurture your bond with your spouse.

You can leave a lasting legacy that will influence future generations and forge close, loving relationships with your family and community by adhering to these values.

As we acknowledge the crucial role fathers play in families and the influence they have on the lives of their children, let's unite to support and uplift them in this important duty. Let's dispel negative gender stereotypes and highlight strong male role models to make the world a more accepting and encouraging place for dads from all backgrounds.

By encouraging a feeling of camaraderie among men and families, we can help make the world a better place for everyone by offering resources and assistance when required. In honor of the special qualities and contributions that fathers provide to their families and communities, let's celebrate fatherhood in all its manifestations. One family at a time, we can work together to create a more loving, caring, and understanding world.